What to Do About a
'BAD BACK'
and
DISC TROUBLE

What to Do About a

'BAD BACK'

and

DISC TROUBLE

by

H. Clements

DRAKE PUBLISHERS

NEW YORK

ISBN 87749-152-6

Published in 1972 by
Drake Publishers Inc.
381 Park Avenue South
New York. New York 10016

Library of Congress Catalog Card Number : 70/175969

CONTENTS

INTRODUCTION

ALTHOUGH disc troubles must have been a problem for many years before, it is only since about 1930 that we have realised the importance of this spinal structure in causing backache, sciatica, and other allied symptoms. Since its recognition the problem seems to have increased, so that now it has become a major one. It is true to say that almost every family may have, or know of, a sufferer, and the term 'slipped disc' is in everyone's vocabulary.

The problem at the present time is huge and growing. It has been estimated that well over a million people suffer through disc troubles, and it can be a particularly crippling complaint. For the individual it means a loss of work and a good deal of suffering. In the acute stage of the trouble it may mean a session in hospital with the possibility of having to wear a corset for some time afterwards. It may only mean a period of bed rest at home, but this may be a matter of weeks and even months.

At best it means a considerable decrease in the physical efficiency of the individual, and a loss of working hours for the community. It is no respector of persons; the young and the old may suffer, and sometimes the ones who feel they are the most fit find themselves flat on their backs. One can, of course, get considerable help from various forms of treatment which may extend from manipulation to surgery, but it is peculiarly a condition where the individual may have to practice his own personal sense of responsibility to make full recovery possible.

These facts make one realise that prevention is the only real answer to the problem, and here again it is very much up to the individual to play his own part in the procedure. The problem is mainly one of body mechanics and posture, and these have to be understood if we are able to get disc troubles into their proper perspective.

In the course of evolution man has acquired an erect position for his body, and with it some problems for the spine in conforming to it. The spinal column, in particular, had to undergo many changes, and the ones which changed it from the horizontal to the vertical position demanded a good deal of adaptation. In changed entirely the balance of the body, altering its support from four to two supports, at the same time placing greater strains on both the muscular and nervous systems. It also completely changed the function of weight-bearing, since the spine, no longer in the horizontal plane, found itself balancing its weight in the vertical one. Thus, the spine, once functioning as a beam now had to adapt itself to the disadvantages of becoming a pillar, in which the spinal discs were detrimentally placed. Now, the whole of the weight of the head and the upper part of the body had to be transmitted through them, in addition to which they had to absorb the shocks which were now more obviously directed towards the brain and the nervous system. The body had constantly to struggle against the forces of gravity, a top heavy mass with the inadequacy of only two supports.

In addition to the changes which evolution had brought about in the human body, there were also environmental changes to which it had to adapt itself. For centuries man had roamed the earth using his limbs, his muscles, and his joints to their full capacity; walking over rough ground, climbing trees, and every other kind of natural excercise kept his body strong and vigorous, helping in the development of a flexible, powerful spine. But with the coming of civilised life much of this was bound to change. With the development of transport, the institution of mechanical aids, and the invention of labour saving appliances, there remained little need for the natural exercise that was the lot of the more primitive person. But the body can no more do without exercise than it can do without food, and thus began the troubles which arose as a result of the lack of it. In particular the muscles, the joints and associated structures were bound to be affected, and with this came the weakened spinal column upon which constant and varied movements depend.

Whatever the answer may be, there can be little doubt that there is no real substitute for physical exercise, and when it cannot be had as a part of everyday life then efforts must be made to provide it in some kind of planned programme. The widespread prevalence of disc troubles makes this imperative. We have no other options. Whatever may be claimed for drugs and other methods of treatment for other complaints, the fact remains that when it comes to the afflictions of the joints and muscles, prevention is better than cure, and this means that they should all be used—if not, then at least kept in good condition. It is important therefore that the individual should know something about their construction and function so that he will be able to make the best use of his time and effort in being able to choose the right exercises and, equally important, to apply them properly

To fulfil these requirements is the chief aim of this book, which is written after a great many years of experience in managing established disc troubles, with the thought that so much might have been done in the preventive stages. Curiously enough, many people have a reluctance to what one might term artificial exercise, i.e. set movements that are designed to keep the discs, muscles, and joints in good condition. But for those who are living a citified life with no proper exercise there is no other choice. It is rather a question of "exercise or else".

Finally, important as exercise is, we must not overlook the fact that there can be no real health or strength in the structures of the body unless there is proper nutrition. This means that the body must be supplied with adequate and suitable food. Generally speaking, this should be fairly easy in these days of abundance, but as we point out it takes a little knowledge of both the quantitive and protein value in foods, and we have taken the trouble to say a few wise words about it.

CHAPTER ONE

THE SYMPTOMS OF DISC TROUBLES

IN spite of popular opinion to the contrary, disc troubles do not just spring out of the blue; there are usually warning signs that should never go unheeded. When people are carefully questioned about them, it will usually be found that there have been back symptoms which give a clear indication that all is not well in the spine. The trouble may not amount to much more than discomfort in the lower back and perhaps some aching in the lower limbs. Such discomfort may be rather more troublesome after a job that calls for back bending, or it may be that it will be more noticeable in the morning when rising from bed. Sometimes it will show itself after sitting in an easy chair when the back is held in a rounded-out position. These early signs of disc trouble may persist for months, and perhaps years, without receiving any real attention and it is only when the first sharp attack of pain occurs that the individual is made to feel that something must be done.

The sharp pain of disc trouble is usually a frightening experience. It may be something like an electric shock that goes right through the lower body, and if the sciatic nerve is involved, down the leg. It lasts only for a matter of seconds but it is followed by a muscular spasm that will pull the spine to one side and make movement and bending practically impossible. In the acute stage the patient may rest until the pain has eased but even after that there may be a deep aching sensation and considerable muscular stiffness that will interfere with normal activity.

Coughs and Colds and Disc troubles

It is not an uncommon experience to find that the acute attack often coincides with a cold, especially with one where there have been heavy bouts of coughing. Few people realise that a cough is a kind of an explosive effort that expends a good deal of its force through the lower back, and places a very definite strain on the muscles, ligaments and discs of that region. In addition, it is believed that when one is suffering from a cold, changes take place in many parts of the system not merely in the air passages, and it is possible that the water content of the discs may be increased at such a time making them much more liable to strain. Whatever the reason, there is no doubt that it is a wise thing at such a time not to indulge in strenuous activities. Working off a cold by vigorous exercise is a foolish procedure which many people have discovered to their own cost.

Bed Rest and Operations

After a longish period of bed rest, due perhaps to some kind of illness, great care should be taken to save the spine from strain in the early days after rising. It is well known that whereas in days gone by people were kept on their backs for considerable periods, the present day trend is to get them up on their feet as soon as possible. The reason for this is because such inactivity is really very weakening and does not conduce to a good circulation and drainage of the body. This, in itself, is a very good thing, but there is still need to exercise care when returning to normal activities.

This is particularly true after operations and if there are any signs of backache following such a procedure, great care should be taken to gently exercise the spine so as to get it into normal shape, and to make sure that there is no undue strain on the spinal discs. During the convalescent stage a few corrective exercises directed to the mobilisation of the spinal structures can be most rewarding, and a great help in restoring physical efficiency.

Distribution of Pains

We have already intimated how closely the spinal discs are associated with the important nerve trunks which supply the whole of the body and it is not difficult to understand how any irritation to them may give rise to all kinds of vague aches and pains over many areas of it, sometimes simulating other forms of disease so that differentiation may be difficult. Disc trouble in the neck may give rise to pain in the shoulders, arms and other parts of the upper body while in the lumbar region of the spine, the pains may be distributed over the lower parts of the body and the legs and feet.

The term neuritis may be applied to the pains that affect the arms and hands, whilst the term sciatica, the most usual form of nerve affection applies to those pains in the legs or feet. Indeed, sciatica is most frequently caused by some disorder of the spinal discs and any vague pains in the legs and the feet should call for some investigation of the lumbar spine.

Effects of Disc Trouble on the General Health.

There is no complaint more fatiguing than some form of back trouble, and if it continues over a long period it is more than likely to undermine the general health. In order to get relief from it many people indulge themselves in pain-killers, such as aspirin, and preparations containing phenacetin. The former may upset the stomach and digestion and the latter will cause trouble with the kidneys. In this indirect way disc trouble may be an unsuspected cause of much ill health.

Losing Precious Time

One cannot repeat too often that it is in the early stages of back trouble that so much can be done to ensure complete recovery. But many people lose precious time by thinking that the trouble will right itself; in most cases it will do nothing of the kind and the most usual thing for it to do is to go from bad to worse. A recent investigation in the United States showed that some people may wait for as long as a year before obtaining treatment for a backache and this gives one some idea of how established a complaint can become.

When a Back Injury needs Attention

When a person sustains an injury that affects the spine it is usual for him to rest until the acute pains have subsided. How long this will be naturally depends upon the seriousness of the injury, but what is really important is that recovery should not be considered to be complete until the spine may be put through its full movements without causing pain and discomfort. Unfortunately, this rule is not always followed, and it is not unusual to meet people who date their backache back to an injury which started the trouble.

In all such injuries the discs have to bear the brunt of the strain and the danger of not overcoming the effects completely is that it may leave a focal point for the development of rheumatism and arthritis. It is a well known fact that many cases of arthritis have started after an injury and the starting point for it is likely to be in the cartilaginous tissue of which, of course, the spinal discs are formed.

No one should be completely satisfied that an injury, especially to the back, has been properly managed if the spine is still suffering from vague symptoms and is definitely limited in its movements. So much trouble in the future will be prevented if this fact is kept in mind.

Slips and Falls in Childhood and the Spinal Discs

Children and drunken men are sometimes said to fall without injury but this is not always true of children. The fact is that a child may fall and injure himself without the injury being apparent. But it may be there just the same. This is particularly true of the spinal discs. Of course, all the tissues in the young body are soft and more pliable and less likely to damage than in an older person but they may be injured just the same. For that reason a fall during childhood should be treated with real concern until one is more than satisfied that full recovery from it has been made. The fall may put the spine off balance so that extra strain is suffered by one or more of the discs and in time this may lead to bad posture and the accompanying backache in later life.

Sometimes children may have quite severe falls without informing the parents, possibly because they may have been up to some mischief and loth to let the parents know about it. Unexplainable disc troubles may arise in this way, although oftimes adults will recall such occurrences. After an injury the spine should be put fully through all its movements to make quite sure that the discs are functioning normally. This will often save a great deal of trouble in later life.

CHAPTER TWO

WHAT YOU SHOULD KNOW ABOUT THE SPINE

IT is sometimes surprising to find that most people know so little about the various parts of their own bodies. Take, for example, the spine. It is very doubtful if an ordinary member of the public ever thinks about its structure or its function referring to it mainly as the backbone. Yet a modicum of knowledge about its general make-up and the vital part which it plays in all the essential movements of the body would be of the greatest help in enabling the individual to make the best use of it and to preserve it in its full integrity into old age. When disc and other spinal troubles develop, they limit full movement, incapacitate the whole of the system and undermine the general health.

Structure of the Spine

If we could view the spine from the front and the back it would resemble a pyramid, broadening quite regularly toward its base. If we had a side view of it we should see that it resembles a long S curve and at the back of it we should recognise the jutting out bones that we can feel with our fingers when we run them down the back of the body. We should also observe that the spinal column is much thicker than many people would imagine, indeed, it is as thick as it is wide, and, again, to many people's surprise, occupies about one-half of the diameter of the body from front to back. The reason for the pyramidal shape and the central position of the spine is to give it the necessary great strength for the support of the whole body. And the S-shaped curve of it has developed in order to sustain the bodily weight when in the upright position.

In order that the spine should be a highly flexible organ

certain elements have to enter into its construction, and Nature has met this need with great ingenuity. It consists mainly of a series of bones with discs set between almost all of them. They number 33 in all and are made up as follows: Seven vertebrae which compose the neck or the cervical region and which supports the head, assisting also in the partial support of the shoulders, arms and the chest; twelve dorsal vertebrae, to which the ribs are attached and which help to form the cavity of the chest for the support and protection of the heart, lungs and some of the abdominal organs; five lumbar vertebrae, the largest of the whole series which are mainly involved in weight-bearing and flexibility; five sacral vertebrae which are all fused together and form what is called the sacrum; and finally, the four small vertebra, named as the coccyx and are said to be the remnants of the long lost tail.

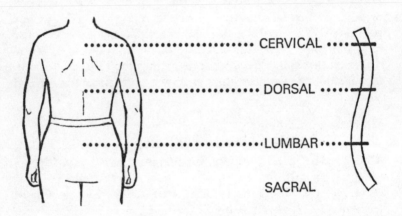

The individual vertebra consist of a rounded body, with various bony processes and the formation of a neural arch through which the vital spinal cord passes. The solid or body part of the vertebrae are held together by what are known as the discs. These are worth thinking about for a moment because they play a very important part in the normal working of the spine and are, of course, of particular interest to us in the subject which we are discussing.

They consist of a ring of cartilage, the shape of their adjacent bones, and are firmly fixed to the bony surfaces. The discs are attached to the vertebrae by very strong criss cross fibres and the outer part of the disc is quite firm. Inside the disc there is a soft gelatinous substance that is able to move and accommodate the movement and weight-bearing functions of the spine, and at the same time permit the freest possible motion consistent with the limitation of the bones.

The vertebrae and the discs form, therefore, a flexible rod and if we took such a rod in our hands we could manipulate it in all directions, because the discs would act as a ball and socket joint. In the body the spine has to be controlled in its movements by the use of ligaments and muscles. The ligaments are employed to strengthen and reinforce the many joints while the muscles provide the motivating forces. We might, for the sake of simplicity, think of the spinal muscles as a kind of system of guy ropes which support the spinal column of bones and discs and assist them in the various and complicated movements that are being constantly performed in daily life.

Apart from the structures of the spine that are directly concerned with its support and movement we should bear in mind the intimate connection between the spine and the nervous system. The spine houses, of course, the great spinal cord which is the continuation of the brain and through the spinal canals, formed by the grooves in the vertebrae, pass the nerve trunks which arises from the spinal cord. These nerve trunks are closely associated with the discs and the pains occurring as a result of disc troubles may be caused by the irritation of these nerve trunks. When the discs are in normal condition they keep the vertebrae together but apart and thus protect the vital nerve pathways.

Like all other parts of the body the spine is supplied with blood vessels which maintain the circulation of blood through its tissues. A normal circulation, as we know, is essential to life and this is particularly true of the spine and its nervous system. To keep up the circulation it is vitally important that there should be movement in the joints and the muscles which gives the stimulus to the flow of blood in the veins. It has been truly said that movement is life.

B

The Functions of the Spine

The chief function of the spine, apart from the protection which it gives to the spinal cord and the nervous system, is to act as a support for the body, to assist in the distribution and the bearing of the body weight and to promote and control body movements. The supporting function of the spine is very important seeing that it has to constantly accommodate itself to the various loads, of the head, chest and pelvis and to adjust them in all the complicated movements that may affect them. And withal it has to maintain the upright balance of the body against the forces of gravity.

Weight-bearing, support and balance are very important functions for the spine to fulfil as we realise at once when we think of the head itself. Not in itself an inconsiderable weight it has to be supported on the top of the spine and it has to be maintained in balance no matter what bodily movement may take place when in the upright position. Unless the spine is in a condition to properly fulfil this function then the whole of the system may suffer. The body will be put under strain and a great deal of nervous energy will be expended in trying to restore lost balance.

Balance, is of course the primary requisite of an efficient spine and is dependent upon the flexibility of the tissues and joints. When flexibility is lost, in any small measure, support and weight-bearing will be impaired, and the spine, as the central controlling influence, will fail in its main functions. This failure will be shown in the poor posture of the body when the weight of the head and upper body will tend to distort the figure, a characteristic that can be seen in so many people.

The Spine and the Nervous System

Many people think of the spine as being merely a kind of backbone and do not realise how closely it is associated with the nervous system. They may suffer from all kinds of aches and pains in various parts of the body, in the muscles of the back and abdomen, in the hands and feet, and other parts of the limbs and sometimes in the various regions of the head. While they may be inclined to think that they may have a 'touch of rheumatism' the fact is that their origin is in the spine.

These aches and pains arise in most cases from irritation of the nerve trunks which, as we mentioned before, pass through the spinal canals. As long as the spine is kept in normal condition there is no likelihood of any interference with these nerve trunks, but changes in the spine, which may be brought about by injury, rigidity of various areas, thinning of the discs, bad posture and so on, will bring in its train compression and consequent irritation of the nerve trunks leading to the various parts of the body and this in its turn will be the cause of the vague aches and pains.

The muscles of the body may be affected in this way and this is the reason why one may find that there are many tender spots in the muscles of the back. If the nerve irritation continues it may cause weakness or spasms in the muscles and this may lead to weakness in the hands and feet. When people suffer from tingling of the hands and feet we may be sure that the spinal nerves are irritated, and of course, when sciatica is present the irritation comes from interference with the lumbar nerves.

Whenever such symptoms are experienced attention should be directed to the condition of the spine and as little time as possible spent in trying to alleviate the aches and pains with pain-killers. The irritation to the nerve trunks is of a mechanical nature and we must endeavour to make the spine into a more efficient instrument if the troubles are to be overcome.

The Lifeline of the Body

It cannot be stressed too often that the spine is the lifeline of the body. We believe that it is in many ways the most neglected domain of the body and that through such neglect a great many ailments occur that would not arise if the importance of the spine was more clearly expressed. We should not forget that in assuming the upright position of the body, as man did rather late in his evolution, he placed a great strain upon the vertebral column, and even at this stage of his development it may be true to say that the spine has not been fully adapted to its environment. With the constant changing of this environment, the use of the car and other methods of transport, it may well be that unless we consciously help the spine in its adaptation processes it may never adjust itself.

It has been estimated that in this country alone there may be something like a million people who suffer from infirmities of the back in which the spinal discs are involved in a breakdown. This obviously places a great strain on the affected individual but it also means a great loss in working hours to the community. It is sometimes overlooked at the present time that in so many occupations the physical efficiency of the individual is the greatest asset, and this, in effect, means a mobile and flexible spine.

You are as Young as Your Spine

One of the first signs of advancing age is the stooping spine. Another, of course, is the diminution of one's height. In both cases the discs of the spine are directly involved. When one is young and the discs are resilient they can return to their normal position after strain; when one is beginning to feel the ravages of age the discs no longer retain their elasticity and tend to become fixed in certain positions. As the body tends to bend forward during the daily occupation the shape of the discs may be gradually altered so that it is more difficult to regain an upright position. Hence the tendency to stoop. This position creeps on stage by stage. The head is held forward and the curve in the neck is changed. The shoulders are rounded and the chest cramped. There is a much greater strain across the lower back and the discs in the lumbar region of the spine become wedge-shaped. The old age picture is being irrevocably drawn.

When it becomes noticeable that a person is not as tall as in earlier days we may be sure that age is taking its toll and that the tissues of the body are hardening and drying out. This is literally true of the spinal discs. The shrinkage in height is in direct ratio to the shrinkage of the discs and with it there is a lack of mobility of the body as a whole, particularly of the movements in which the spine is directly concerned.

While it is true, of course, that the oncoming of age is inevitable it is also true to say that a great deal may be done to mitigate its drawbacks and infirmities if the spine is kept flexible by suitable measures that will ensure the normal condition of the spinal discs.

CHAPTER THREE

THE SPINAL DISCS

LET us now take a little closer look at the spinal discs and their relation to the spine and the rest of the body. They represent about a quarter of the whole length of the spine and they are thicker in the parts of it where there is freer movement, such as in the neck and the lumbar region. In the dorsal area, where the ribs are attached to the spine and where there is little movement they are rather thinner. Apart from the fact that they hold the spinal bones together, they also keep them separated so as to protect the nerve trunks, and they do to some extent act as shock absorbers. It stands to reason that if the spine consisted only of bone many of the shocks and jars to which the body is constantly subjected would be transmitted direct to the brain and would in serious cases cause concussion. For that reason young people, whose discs are full and healthy, are much better able to withstand falls and other forms of violence than older people whose discs are thinned and hardened.

What Happens When they are Injured

A normal disc can stand quite of lot of strain and, of course, is subjected to it in the course of ordinary activity. Naturally like any other part of the human body it may be damaged by the use of excessive force. It is unlikely that this would occur in the course of ordinary activities and it is to falls and other accidents that we must look for such injuries. The discs in the neck and the lower back where there is the greatest amount of movement are the parts of the spine where we are most likely to find the damaged discs. In recent years many people have suffered from injuries to the discs of the

neck due to car accidents and in the United States the term
'whiplash' injury has been devised to describe such damage.
But any violent movement that jerks the neck will have the
same effect in damaging the tissues of this area and lead to the
symptoms which may follow.

Apart, then from the strain that will take place in the surrounding ligaments and muscles, when violence is applied to
the spine, we have to consider its effect upon the disc itself.
In the more serious case the disc may be herniated or rup-
tured. The term 'hernia' applied to any part of the body
means protrusion, and this is what happens with the discs.
The outer part of it is breached and some of the softer gelatinous matter protrudes. The amount of pain and difficulty
which it will produce will depend upon its location. Because
of its proximity to the nerve trunks the protrusion may be
merely an irritating influence, or it may cause an actual
pressure on them, and this, of course, will lead to severe pain,
such as may be experienced in sciatica when the injured disc
is in the lumbar region. Fortunately such a serious injury to
the disc is a fairly rare occurrence; in the majority of cases
it is strain rather than an actual breakdown that has occurred.

The So-called Slipped Disc

For some reason or other the term 'slipped disc' has been
applied to almost any pain that is felt in the back and this has
led to many mistaken ideas about the condition. It is easy to
imagine that anything separating two bones might slip but
when we remember that the disc is firmly anchored to each
bone and well supported by powerful ligaments we see how
absurd the notion is. If this were so, then even if it could be
easily replaced it could just as easily slip out again. The term
slipped disc is gradually being abandoned and it is more than
likely that it will be forgotten in the near future.

Nutrition and the Health of the Discs

It is rather unfortunate that when specific troubles arise in
the body, like for example, the case of the intervertebral disc,
people are apt to forget the relationship between any weakness
of the body and nutrition. Yet it is true to say that nutrition

is the basis of life and we forget this fact at our peril. There is no doubt that when the nutrition of the system is impaired every part of it will suffer in some way. Our nutrition depends of course on the food that we eat and assimilate and if there should be any deficiency in that respect then a high standard of health and resistance to disease cannot be maintained. From this standpoint whenever bodily health is below par there is an added danger where the discs are concerned and they are liable to break down more quickly under any kind of strain. One should remember that assisting in the support of the body as they do and with the constant weight-bearing of its various parts any nutritional disorders like obesity can produce that extra strain which may prove the last straw.

Discs and Bodily Age

We must be aware that as age advances and the signs of it become apparent, the greying of the hair, the drying of the skin and such other noticeable differences between age and youth, the condition of the discs will change also. They will tend to lose their high water content and to have less elasticity in them so that under weight-bearing strain they may become slightly reduced in depth. This will cause no particular difficulty but it should remind those who are at such a stage of life that discretion in violent exercises is the course of wisdom.

Discs and Backache

While it is true that backache occurs with practically every case of lesioned discs, there are other cases of backache that are not due to this cause. If we except backache that may be associated with serious disease states, then it is true to observe that the measures which are employed for the prevention of disc trouble are also invaluable for the prevention of backache, so that the distinction between them is not as great as one may be inclined to suppose. What we must have in mind at all times, when we are thinking about any kind of spine trouble, is that the whole of it is involved no matter how local the immediate trouble seems to be. This is especially true of exercise and is a viewpoint that should always be kept in mind.

Rheumatism and Arthritis and the Spinal Discs

Both these forms of disease affect the locomotor system of the body in which the joints and the muscles play the major part, and obviously this means that the discs must be affected in some ways. These diseases are the most widespread of all, and it is estimated that almost fifty per cent of people over sixty years of age suffer from them. Often starting quite early in life, the changes which they bring about in the various tissues of the system are of course, not felt until later in life when they are fully developed.

Rheumatism affects particularly the muscles and this tends to limit their action in the movement of the joints which deteriorate when they are not fully employed. The cartilaginous tissue of the joints become involved and when changes take place in them the first stage of arthritis has started. The discs of the spine are, of course, composed of cartilage and they share in the general arthritic disease which sooner or later will spread to them. When this happens the changes in the tissues will so weaken the discs that they will no longer be able to carry out their weight-bearing and supporting tasks and will tend to lose their elasticity and become very much thinner as may be shown on X-rays. In some cases the discs will lose their normal resistance and prolapse. Then, of course, the vertebrae may be brought nearer together and some pressure may be exerted on the nerve trunks. These are chronic and irremediable cases when they enter this stage because it is impossible to regenerate cartilage tissue when it has been destroyed.

The important thing to bear in mind if there is rheumatism and/or arthritis in the system is to avoid as much as possible straining efforts which would place pressure upon the spinal discs. Such a person must be counselled to do things moderately and to live within his physical capacity. On the other hand, this should not be taken as a counsel of despair, particularly in the early stages of these forms of disease. One should remember that joints and muscles, and incidentally the discs and other cartilaginous tissues, need movement to keep up their nutrition and to remove their waste products. Exercise, correctly taken, is therefore a very important preventive measure in both rheumatism and arthritis and the same measures which will help to keep the discs in good condition will be most helpful in preventing these diseases and in arresting their development when they are established.

CHAPTER FOUR

THE URGENT NEED FOR PREVENTION

THE old axiom that prevention is better than cure will never be refuted. It is easier, it is safer and it is less costly in every way. It can never be repeated too often when one is thinking about disc and back troubles. While no one would be so dogmatic as to say that prevention will always succeed in these cases the chances are so good that it is folly not to try. Nothing will be lost and everything stands to be gained.

Proper Use of the Body

The spine is the great determinant of all the body's activities. It remains the fundamental basis for all the various bodily structures. The strength of arms and legs depends upon their closeness of association with the strongest parts of the spine. The great muscles binding the pelvis and legs which extend deep into the trunk depend on the strength of the lower spine, and in all the activities in which the body is engaged the strength of the spine is of paramount importance.

The body may be used rightly or wrongly; good habits are as easy to establish as bad ones, but to be sure that such habits are in conformity with the body's best interest we must be aware of what we are doing. The best yardstick for our guidance is the position of the spine. Our posture must be easy so that the balance of the spine is preserved, and whatever movement we do we must try to be aware of the flexibility of the spine. We may be sure that when we are unable to maintain balance in the body when walking, standing, sitting and generally moving about, the cause of it will be found in the uneven pull of the muscular guy ropes of the back. Impaired functioning of the spinal discs results, and these are the main factors to be considered. Their rectification will help in restoring physical efficiency.

Occupations That are Hazardous

Some occupations throw a good deal of strain on the spinal discs. Standing and sitting in bad positions for long periods may tend to change the shape of the discs and render them liable to give trouble. Car seats that do not properly support the spine may often lead to a strained back with the disc as the main focal point of the trouble. No one can, of course, give precise instructions as to how these positions may be avoided, but if the general ideas which we have described, relating to the structure and function of the spine, are borne in mind it is possible for the individual to work out for himself corrective positions.

In many occupations and in sport and games there is a tendency to use one hand and arm and one side of the body more than the other, and this can upset the balance of the spine and disturb the uniformity of the muscular guy ropes of the spine; if it is not possible to reverse the position in the work or the pastime then exercises should be performed to equalize the balance of the spinal muscles.

The Weekend Gardener

The weekend gardener needs special notice in relation to disc troubles. It is common practice to sit in an office most of the week and then at the weekend undertake some vigorous gardening work. The bending of the back in digging and planting, and other jobs that have to be done, throws a real strain on the back and oft-times the result is a persistent backache. This is generally a pointer to the fact that the discs are under strain and some thought should be given to a few corrective exercises.

And it may be an indication also that not enough attention is given to the way in which the weekend tasks are carried out. We think far more about the use of our tools than the use of the body. Yet, in the last analysis the body is a mechanical instrument, based on the lever system. The three lever systems are found in the arrangement of the muscles, tendons and bones, examples of which one can easily find for oneself. With a little ingenuity in this way much better use may be made of the body and far less strain placed upon it.

Lifting and Straining

Many cases of back and disc troubles are due to lifting and straining, and the fact that they are steadily on the increase makes one realise that more attention should be paid to these causative factors. Everybody must, at some time, do some kind of lifting and with it there is always the possibility of strain. Even in the home there is the moving of furniture, the lifting of children and other chores that place the back and discs at risk. The same thing applies in many occupations, but it is not always in those where really heavy lifting has to be done that damage may occur. In those cases there has been much more preliminary training and the muscles and other structures are able to meet the strain. It is far more likely to happen when a person is suddenly called upon to do some lifting to which he is not accustomed and which he attempts to do without giving it any previous thought.

There are certain rules about lifting and using one's strength that should be carefully learnt if trouble is to be avoided. One of the most important, and indeed the simplest of these rules, is to always remember to bend the knees whenever one is going to make a heavy lift. The interesting thing about this is that it is practically impossible to strain the back when the knees are bent, as anyone can easily prove for himself. As a matter of fact, it is a good plan at all times when one is standing to let the knees slightly bend or relax because by so doing the strain is taken off the muscles, and is thrown on to the ligaments of the joints, and as ligaments do not contract and relax as muscles do, they do not tire. It is interesting also to notice that when the knees are relaxed in this way there is far less strain on the back muscles even when one is just standing and not attempting to lift a weight. In time the bent knees become a habit which is a great safeguard so far as the back and the discs are concerned.

Another important rule, that should always be observed, is that the feet should, when one is standing for long periods or doing some kind of lifting, be slightly turned inward. By so doing the weight of the body comes on to the outside of the feet where it is most easily borne, and in addition to this, by holding the feet in this position, the pelvis is placed in a much more invulnerable one. One can readily demonstrate this for oneself and it will be noticed that as the feet are turned inward so the abdomen tends to be pulled slightly upwards.

On the other hand, it will be noticed that the protruding abdomen goes with the out-turned feet, and also, of course when the feet are in this position then the weight of the body falls on the inside of the feet. The inside of the feet are the springlike parts which aid in the act of propulsion, so that the whole of the movement of the body is impeded in some way by the wrong position of the feet Finally, outsplayed feet will throw strain on the back and discs by interfering with the normal posture of the body.

Another point which should always be kept in mind when using the body is to remember that it is when the spine is in rotation that it is most easily strained. So long as the movement is just bending forward and backward there is a fairly equal pull on the muscles of the back and strain is less likely; it is when one is turned slightly to one side and a lift or a strenuous movement is made that the damage is likely to be done. For example, sitting at a desk and leaning sideways to shut a drawer or pushing up a window with a sideways movement with the spine off centre are the kind of movements that may well bring disaster. The muscles of the back may contract violently to the one side straining the discs in the process.

Even the lifting of some light object, perhaps a coal scuttle, may strain the muscles of the spine if the body is turned slightly to one side during the effort. This may be obviated to a certain extent if the knees are consciously relaxed, but whenever the spine is in torsion there is a real possibility that the strain will fall on the discs and the other structures producing some trouble.

Standing and Sitting

Those who may have to stand for long periods at a time

should make a point of adopting a stance that will throw the least amount of strain upon the back. It is helpful to bear in mind that when we stand in the stand-easy position we are allowing the muscles to relax and for the weight to come onto the ligaments. All the joints of the body are held together by ligaments and there is a provision in some of them, like for example, the hip joint where the ligaments are so arranged that they can take the place of the muscles when we are in the stand-easy position. Allow the pelvic area to fall slightly forward and the ligament will automatically lock the hip joint and the position can be held without further effort. Another point to remember about the standing position is that the body is never completely stationary. It is gently swaying all the time, and it is only when we stand consciously rigid that we do away with this swaying movement. This is a very tiring thing to do. So when we are standing it is a good thing to let the body sway very slightly like a tree in a breeze; it is surprising how relaxing this movement can be.

A good deal of strain may be thrown on the spine if we sit in an awkward position. Sitting in a soft chair with the lower back rounded out puts a real strain on the lumbar discs and may weaken the muscles. Leaning to one side when in the sitting position, as when writing at a desk, may in time alter the shape of the discs, especially when this is done in early life, as, for instance, in the case of a school child. The straight-back chair, which tends to keep the lumbar inward curve, is probably the best sitting position. The car seats should be so arranged that the lumbar region is supported with its slightly inward curve and not allowed to round out into the back of the seat. Unless the lumbar curve is well supported when sitting up in bed, the position may well bring on a backache from a strained spine.

The Importance of Strong Flexible Feet

The connection between the feet and the spine is sometimes overlooked. We have already pointed out that the position of the feet when standing is very important and we should stress the fact that the condition of the feet themselves is equally important. The feet have to bear the weight of the whole body and this should be equally distributed between the two. In many cases this is not so, one foot bearing more weight than the other. Occasionally this unevenness of weight carrying may be due to a fallen arch in the one foot which may tend to upset the balance of the spine also. The feet also act as shock absorbers but if the arches are fallen or rigid this important function will not be properly carried out and, in consequence, the shocks will be transmitted to the spine, where the discs will have to receive and absorb them. Strong, flexible feet, with good power of propulsion are one of the most valuable assets which help to keep the spine in balance and the whole body in general fitness.

Bed Strain

Owing to the widespread number of disc troubles thousands of sufferers have had to support their beds with boards. This is done mainly to stop the bed from sagging. After a bed has been in use for some years it tends to lose its resistance and this makes it very difficult for a person to turn over on it without straining the back muscles. As a rule the boards are not used until an attack has been suffered, but this is rather late in the day if one is thinking in terms of prevention. If the bed shows any sign of sagging it should be renewed or fitted with a firm board to take up the strain.

Holiday Beds

A few nights spent on a bed that sags will often provoke a backache and that has been the experience of many people who have been away on holidays and slept on sagging beds. It is not easy, of course, to suggest a remedy for this sort of thing but to be aware of the danger may help one to avoid it. It reminds one of a woman who used, every few months, to visit her parents in the country and who came back to her home suffering from backache after every visit. A change to a firmer bed in her parents' home, and the abandonment of the old feather-filled one, prevented any further attacks. If we remember that we spend a third of our lives in bed and that during that time we go through quite a few movements, changing from one position to another, the importance of a firm surface is at once apparent.

Sports and Games

In some sports and games one part of the body is used more than another and if a strain should result from this it will make itself felt in the spine. Using the right arm and shoulder more than the left, and vice versa, as, for example, in tennis, can lead to over-development on the one side of the body and upset the balance of the spinal muscles. This in time may lead to a lop-sided posture which will throw a definite strain on the spinal discs and this may be the reason why we sometimes read of an athlete, who is thought to be in first class physical condition, going down with disc trouble. The remedy for this kind of thing is for the adoption of corrective exercise to balance up the muscular system.

Violent exercise, allied to sports and games, may not show any adverse effects during the active stage when it is being carried on, but that is not to say that adverse effects may not be seen in later life. As we have seen the spinal discs are shock absorbers with obviously a limited capacity. The shocks which they may sustain from violent falls and personal encounters may easily leave some damaged tissues in the spinal discs which in later life provides a suitable focal point for the development of such complaints as rheumatism and arthritis. Given a family predisposition to these troubles, the risk is quite considerable.

The Need for Proper Preparation

Preliminary preparation should be undertaken before indulging in any kind of vigorous exercise, including, of course, sports and games. The central theme of such training should be the spinal column and its vitally important structures. First of all, it should be seen that the muscles of the spine are well developed, and equally as important, that they should be well balanced. This will mean that with an even pull of the guy ropes of the back the pressure on the intervertebral will be equalised. Any rigid area of the spine should

c

be carefully mobilised since a lack of flexibility is probably the greatest danger the spine can suffer.

All the movements of the spine should be carefully tested to make sure that they are not limited in any way, and it is particularly important to see that the rotation movements of the spine are in normal condition, since it is, generally speaking, when it is moving in this way that breakdowns occur. A week or so of training, with these essential points in mind, will often save a lot of trouble in the future.

Exercise: The Right Attitude

Exercise devoted to the development of the body started with the strong man idea of Sandow and those who followed him. For a long time the main idea was the development of the muscular system. No doubt this was beneficial, but it omitted an important phase of such exercise that should never be overlooked: that the integrity of the joints of the body should have prior attention, especially those of the spinal column, since in the last analysis unless joints are operating normally the muscles will lose their efficiency. Tennis elbow is a good case in point: unless the joint of the elbow is adjusted no amount of exercise or treatment will restore the function of the adjacent muscles.

CHAPTER FIVE

RECOVERING FROM
DISC TROUBLES

MANY people go for long periods suffering from vague pains in the back without doing very much about it. They are inclined to think of them as a kind of discomfort that has to be borne, and it may well be that a medical examination has not revealed any definite cause for such complaints, and the argument for doing nothing about it may appear to be reinforced. The saying that the patient's backache gives the doctor a headache may have some truth in it.

But then, quite suddenly, the whole picture changes. A heavy straining movement, or, sometimes a very simple light twisting effort may cause acute pain and distress, and the patient is obliged to seek relief by rest. It is too late in the day, then to think about what the causative factor was or what might have been done to prevent it. There can be little doubt that in the majority of these cases the spinal disc or discs have been involved.

If the pain is not too severe and the muscle spasm easily reducible then manipulative treatment may afford considerable relief, but if this is not possible then the sufferer will have to stay in bed until the acute pains have subsided. A firm surface to the bed is absolutely necessary and various positions should be assumed until one is found that gives relief. The application of hot applications over the area where the muscles are in spasm is most helpful and is one of the best ways of comforting the sufferer.

When the acute pain has passed, and the muscle spasm has been reduced, it may be possible to hasten recovery by manipulative treatment, but the next best thing if this is not available or desirable are carefully graduated exercises to relieve the congestion and to restore the normal movements of the affected parts. Experience has shown that the best three movements to start with are as follows:

Lie face downwards. Place a cushion under the chest to elevate the upper part of the body. Hold this position for a few minutes and then add another cushion elevating the upper body still higher. Hold this position for a few minutes, perhaps a little longer than before. Then add another cushion as before. The position will be that the upper part of the body is well elevated and the lower part of the spine will be put into extension. The individual may help this by endeavouring to let the lumbar part of the back relax on the surface of the bed. The position should be held until it begins to get uncomfortable and then the cushions removed one by one, allowing the body to gradually resume the level position.

Second Movement: Lie flat on the back. Bring one knee upwards until you are able to reach it with the hands. Interlace the fingers around the knee and pull the knee up as far as possible on the chest. Then allow the arms to straighten, still holding the knee and then press with the knee against the hands. Relax and lower the leg and then do the same with the other knee. This movement will mobilise the lower lumbar vertebrae, free up the pelvic joints and also stretch the ligaments and the spinal discs.

Third Movement: Lie on your side with the lower hand under the side of the face. Stretch out fully the lower leg. Now bend the upper leg at the knee and allow the knee to fall forward. Then reach back as far as possible with the upper arm and shoulder. If this is done correctly it will rotate the spine in the lower part and relax the musculature of the whole spine. Then turn over to the other side and rotate it in the same way.

If it is found to be possible to do these movements without much discomfort then they should be done several times during the day and done a little more vigorously as time goes along. In some ways the floor is probably the best place on which to do them and this plan should be followed as soon

as possible. The other exercises which we shall describe
later on should gradually be adopted.

It is very important to do everything possible to make recovery complete since it is not one of those cases where one
attack confers an immunity for the future. Indeed, it is probably just the reverse. This is particularly true if measures are not adopted for the building up of the strength and
mobility of the whole spine.

Restoring the Integrity of the Spine

When the more acute phase of the attack has been overcome a good deal of thought should be given to the restora-
tion of the integrity of the whole spine. It will be found that
for some time after the attack there may be vague pains
about the body, and, if the sciatic nerve has been affected, the
pain in the leg may remain for some time even after it is possible to return to ordinary occupations. So long as these
symptoms are present one may be quite sure that the spine is
not functioning normally and that some area of it needs special
attention. It should be tested for its normal movement and
any limitation should be corrected. This may involve a good
deal of patience and perseverance but the long term results
will be more than worthwhile. Unless this is done the complaint may go into the chronic stage and continue to harass
the individual's life for a long time; become as some people
despairingly say a lifelong burden.

The Effects of Smoking

Few people associate smoking with disc and back troubles,
yet indirectly it may be a very real contributory factor. Not
all smokers are, of course, heavy coughers but when they are
afflicted in this way the amount of strain which it imposes
on the back, and especially on the spinal discs, is quite astonish-
ing. This fact is sometimes brought to their notice when
they are in the acute stages of attack of back pain. The explosive effect of the cough will be felt directly at the sore
spot in the spine and may give exquisite pain. Many heavy
smokers go through a strenuous bout of coughing when they
arise in the morning and this may make the spine uncom-

fortable for the rest of the day. The same thing may, of course, occur with any kind of coughing and sneezing which accompanies a cold, but at least these are only experienced occasionally whereas the habitual smokers keeps up the coughing and straining every day of his or her life. Whatever the cause of the coughing may be, unless it can be remedied, it will make the recovery from and prevention of disc troubles very much more difficult.

CHAPTER SIX

PREVENTING DISC TROUBLES

FEW people take the trouble to think about their bodies in the way in which they would think about their cars or other mechanical contrivances with which they are concerned. The tendency is to regard the body and its functions mainly along chemical lines; for this reason people turn to drugs whenever they are affected by ill health. Or, attention is centred on the nervous and emotional side of life and their relationship to health and disease. Apart from being influenced in these ways the body is also a mechanical unit, subject to those principles which govern mechanical bodies.

There is a real need, therefore, to look at the body from this standpoint, especially in relation to disc troubles, since in many ways a great deal of the efficiency of the structures which are involved in the mechanical aspect of the body depend upon the health and integrity of these spinal cartilages. With this in mind, one can carry out a very useful physical self-analysis which will be most helpful in discovering weak points of the system and prove a reliable guide in planning preventive measures.

The mirror test is most useful in this respect. Stand unclothed before a full length mirror and observe the general outlines of the body. It is a good plan to turn a couple of times in a circle so that when facing the mirror the body is in its ordinary position. Observe the way the head is carried. Does it tend to tilt to one side? In cases where there is some tension on one side of the upper spine, possibly due to a compressed disc, this tilt may be very noticeable. One should remember that the neck cannot be bent to one side without rotation and so one may get the impression that the head is turned as well as being bent.

Now take notice of the level of the shoulders. Is one shoulder slightly higher than the other? And as with the head, do the shoulders appear to be twisted, giving the impression that one is further forward than the other? With the hands at the sides does it appear that one hand reaches down farther than the other? Or hang a little farther forward or backward?

Observe the hip and pelvic regions. Again, does one side appear to be higher than the other, and also as with the head and shoulders, does the body appear to be twisted? In some cases this is most noticeable, and, as a matter of interest, it is a condition that is oft-times first called to the individual's attention by a tailor or dressmaker.

Notice the position of the knees. Does one knee appear to be bent slightly and to be held slightly ahead of the other? Notice also the muscles of the upper leg, which, in some cases, may show quite a difference in size due to the fact that the weight of the body may be badly distributed and that one limb has been doing more than its fair share of the job.

The condition and position of the feet should be carefully scrutinised. Do they give the impression of being flat and rigid? In what direction are the toes pointing? Are they lying flat on the floor or give the impression of being curled up? A careful inspection of the feet is well worth while since so much depends upon them as far as the general posture of the body is concerned.

The individual is not able, of course, to view his own back but what he has learned from the foregoing observations will give him a most useful guide to its condition. The tilt of the head, if it exists, will warn him that the structures of the upper spine are under tension and that it is more than likely that there may be thinning of the cervical discs which should receive attention. Tension of this kind in the neck muscles may be a contributory factor in headaches and should not be overlooked.

Variations in the shoulder levels will show that there may be some torsion in the spine, most likely in the lumbar region, and there is not much point, of course, of trying to hold the shoulders level until the underlying cause has been corrected. The same holds true of the pelvic twist which may be due to the same cause. What these conditions denote is that the spine is under strain with most of it centred on a disc or discs, and if it is allowed to continue radical compensatory changes will take place in all the structures of the back.

Any abnormal changes which one might note in the muscles of the legs, the position of the knees and the feet will give one some indication that the weight-bearing functions of the body are not working in harmony. When the weight of the body is thrown over on to one side by perhaps a lowering of the hip, or the arch of the foot, the main strain will be felt in the spine which must be adjusted to maintain the upright position. It may well be that the tilt of the head, the uneven shoulders and pelvis may be directly related to a fallen arch, which, in the ordinary way, would never be suspected of being the cause, unless we view the subject from the standpoint of body mechanics.

Now turn the body sideways and view the back from that angle. Is the head balanced easily on the top of the spine so that it can perform an easy nodding movement? Is the chin held too high so that it causes a kink in the neck? This is a very common fault from which many people may suffer and which may be the cause of vague pains in the neck, and arm and also be associated with headaches. In time the discs, where the kink is not pronounced, will alter their shape and size.

The side view of the body will give one an idea of the state of the curves of the spine. If the curves in the neck and the lower part of the back are too pronounced then the typical rounded shoulders will be seen. If the muscles of the abdomen are in a weakened condition they will sag forward and this will tend to drag on the lower back and increase the lumbar curve.

Having then discussed some of the positions that may be seen with a poor posture let us think of a body that is well poised and in balance. The side view would show that the curves are evenly developed and not too pronounced. The head will be in easy motion and the chin will be held fairly low, so that no kink will form in the neck. The shoulders and the pelvis will be evenly balanced and the feet will be pointing directly ahead with the arches on both feet well developed.

When the body is balanced in that way the spine, as seen from the back, is perfectly straight and as seen from the side, is formed of moderate curves which permits the equal distribution of weight throughout the structures. The spinal discs will then be in the most favourable position to carry out their function in cushioning the vertebrae and allowing the spine to go through all its movements with the minimum of strain. When the body is poised in this way, with no strain on any of its parts, its best general health may be assured. Then it may be held fully erect, with all its muscles, ligaments, bones and joints working freely and with all its vital organs properly housed and protected.

To a great extent the avoidance of disc troubles depend on the attainment of a well balanced and properly co-ordinated posture and everything possible must be done to acquire it. It can be definitely stated that as a general rule whenever there may be found some postural defect the spinal discs will be involved, and unless it is corrected the risk of a disc breakdown cannot be ruled out. The posture of the body is fundamental to good body mechanics and like any other kind of machine that operates on mechanical principles any kind of defective structure will disturb its rhythmn and efficiency.

For that reason it is insisted upon that whenever any part of the system is adversely affected in any way it is to the whole body that we must look for proper rectification. In body mechanics we constantly come up against the vicious cycle: that the parts affect the whole, no less than the whole determines the integrity of the parts. And this rule applies with particular emphasis to the spinal discs and the part which they play in the economy of the bodily system.

The Importance of Wholesome Foods

While it is necessary to emphasise the mechanical aspect of disc troubles and the part which defective posture, injuries, strains and other factors play in the development of them, it would be unwise not to take into consideration the nutritional factor and its vital importance in attaining and maintaining the health and resistance of all the structures in the body. It is a factor that may easily be overlooked, especially in disc troubles where the relationship appears, at first sight, to be rather remote. But a more careful consideration of the matter will show that it is something we may neglect at our peril.

Progress in food production, food preservation and food distribution has brought to people many advantages, but on the other hand, there are certain hazards to be encountered unless we are aware of the effects of these changes upon the foods and upon the human himself. In the main most people in civilised countries live in abundance of foods but unless they are informed about the value of the various foodstuffs and use them intelligently they can starve in the midst of plenty. This is largely due to the fact that so many foods have been processed away from their natural state. It is quite possible at the present time to arrange a menu of foods that may satisfy the appetite and at the same time deprive the body of essential food elements.

We all know that certain elements are required to make our foods complete: Protein, carbohydrates (starches and sugars) fats, vitamins and mineral salts, and that these elements, are, of course, organised and balanced in various foods. However, because of the processes which foods have undergone, we are able to arrange our foods so that we may take much more of a particular food element than if we had to obtain it in its natural state. Sugar is a good example. This element has been extracted from various foods and we are able to take it in excessive quantities. The same is true of some starchy foods like white flour and fats and the foods which are made from them.

Now the danger here is that if we use these foods, almost to the exclusion of other foods, and many people do this because they so easily satisfy the appetite, we are living on what is virtually a deficiency diet. It is true that we may add to these foods the other elements and take supplements of vitamins and mineral salts, but that does not completely obviate the problem. Indeed, the ordinary individual's lack of real knowledge in this respect may easily lead to a lack of balancing factors and do more harm than good.

That many people are living on a deficiency diet because of the excessive use of refined foods is now accepted by many nutritional authorities, and the best example of the result of this is the widespread increase of cases of dental caries. The fact that foods that are deficient in essential elements can cause such troubles should not be lost on those who ought to realise that other structures of the body may be affected in very much the same way. In early life, especially when poor nutrition may undermine the structure of the teeth, it is not too difficult to see that structures like the spinal disc may also be adversely affected so that when adult life is reached these essential supporting and weight-bearing parts of the spine may not be capable of performing their full function.

That this may be an important factor in disc troubles should not be overlooked as witness a statement in the PRESS : 'Millions of families are receiving a diet that may be deficient in one or more nutrients, it is suggested by a report recently published by a department of a Health organization.' The important thing to notice about that report is that it says that the diet may be deficient in one or more of its nutrients, because that means that one might be well satisfied, so far as hunger and taste are concerned, and yet not supplying ones body with the full complement of elements necessary for the maintenance of health and the structures of the system.

The truth is that although it is easy to break down foods into their various parts, it is not so easy to restore them to their original state, and yet it is in their original or natural state that foods contain the essential elements in their proper balance. One of the best adjectives that should be applied to food is the word wholesome. 'Promoting physical or moral health' as the dictionary defines it. Wholesome foods should form the major portion of the menu. It should consist of the protein foods like lean meat, fish, eggs and cheese, of the starchy and sugar foods like the wholegrain products and the fruits and honey, with a generous amount of freshly cooked vegetables, salads and fresh fruit, with as little of the refined and processed foods as circumstances will permit.

In this way the system is supplied with all the essential food elements, including vitamins and minerals, and is able to select sufficient of them to build up the structures of the body and thus prevent breakdowns such as spinal disc troubles.

The Planning of the Exercise Programme

Whenever exercise fails to achieve the results desired one may be fairly sure that it has been used in too much of a hit-or-miss fashion. Many people adopt some kind of a system of exercises and exploit it vigorously for a short time and then abandon it. This is not the way to make exercise really effective. It is better to perform a little exercise regularly so as to keep the joints free and the muscles in good tone. It would, if it is possible, be better to plan a daily programme and then make every effort to keep the schedule. If we think of movement as being as essential to the muscles and joints as food is to the digestive system we may see the point of its daily performance.

This is the proper attitude to adopt towards exercise and then it becomes a daily habit which will be just as easy to carry out as any other daily habit that has, by custom, become ingrained in ones consciousness. So far as the prevention of disc troubles are concerned this is a very important recommendation.

Testing Movements to find the Weak Areas of the Spine

The reader who has already applied the mirror test to his posture and observed the points which have been stressed will have some idea as to whether the spine is functioning normally or whether there are certain defects that should receive attention. There are now a few exercises that should be performed, not so much with the idea of developing the muscles or improving the condition of the other structures as with the object of discovering the various limitations to which the spine and its structures may be subject. It is very important to stress this point. Many people undertake certain exercises and then try to do them whilst completely disregarding some weaknesses that may exist in the body. The result probably being that the stronger parts will become stronger, the weaker ones become strained, and the tyro may give up in despair. So it is necessary to stress that in the early stages all the movements should be done with the idea of finding out the weak spots and then by increasing the range of movement gradually eliminate them.

The exercises should be done on a well-carpeted floor, so as to provide a firm resistance to the body, and enough clothes should be discarded to allow free movement of the various parts of it. And one whole attention should be focused on the exercises when they are being performed.

Exercise 1. Lie flat on the back on the floor with the feet anchored under a heavy piece of furniture or a suitable weighty object. Now attempt to bring the body to the sitting-up position. If there is any difficulty in completing this movement raise only the head the upper part of the body and as the strength increases complete the whole movement. This exercise will develop the important abdominal muscles and will stretch the muscles of the spine, thus benefitting the action of the spinal discs.

Exercise 2. Same position on the floor. Draw the heels up to the buttocks. Place the hands firmly on the abdomen holding it down, as it were. Now try to lift the buttocks and the lower spine off the floor. Do not lift the whole of the back; try to confine the movement to the lower spine and the pelvis. This is easier done than described and is a splendid stimulus to the muscles in the region as well as activating the spinal discs.

Exercise 3. Same position. Lace the fingers around the knees and pull them up as near as possible to chest. Keep the head flat on the floor and open the knees as wide as possible. This exercise may be quite difficult at first and it is a question of using patience rather than strain to get the full movement. This is one of the very best exercises to stretch all the lumbar joints, to keep the muscles of the region well toned up and to make sure that the spinal discs are kept in active use. Do not rock the spine; pull the knees well up and stretch as much as you are able to do without strain.

Exercise 4. Now assume the sitting position with the legs stretched out on the floor. Attempt to reach the toes with your fingers. This places strain on the spinal muscles and ligaments and at the same time stretches the hamstring muscles of the legs. It almost directly affects the sciatica nerve so those who have suffered from this complaint must exercise great care in doing this movement. Many middle aged and older people will find this a testing movement and although they should attempt it, it must be done with real caution.

Exercise 5. Stretch out the body so that it is resting on the hands and the toes, with the arms perfectly straight down from the shoulders. Now take one foot forward as far as possible until the knee touches the arm on that side. Return the foot to the original position and then do the same with the other foot. This is one of the most useful of all exercises that brings into play the important structures of the lower back, the pelvis and the hips. It is not an easy exercise to do for many people and when it does present any difficulty it should be cautiously used. It is a testing movement for the hip joints, and when these are limited in movement the exercise should be assiduously practised, but never with undue strain.

Exercise 6. Stand erect. Now rise slightly on the toes and then bend the knees and assume the squatting position. Then let the heels down on the floor still retaining the squatting position. Many people will find the flat-footed position difficult to assume and if a little support is given by placing the hands on a chair or some other object it will make it easier. This is one of the most valuable of exercises; it strengthens the muscles of the legs and will improve the circulation through the lower part of the body. Here, again, if this position has not been assumed for a long time it will prove very difficult, and the individual must be content at first to make an attempt to do it, realising that in time the muscles will be trained to respond more readily to the effort. It has been found that the practice of this position takes the strain off the lower back and that it can be used as a relief for pain that may be felt in that region of the spine. Some orthopaedic surgeons have suggested that if this position was more usually performed it would strengthen the hips and we would be less likely to hear of the broken ones in later life.

The foregoing exercises should be done at least once daily and each one should be performed a few times until one feels slightly tired. It is impossible to say how many times since each individual differs in strength and endurance. And one should remember that in these testing movements it is much more a matter of seeing how the body, and especially the spine, responds rather than just counting up the number of times that they may be done. Also, of course as time goes along and one is able to do them with the least expenditure of thought and energy, the number of times will naturally increase. What is important also is to note the effect of the exercises upon the posture because if they have been done properly there will be a marked improvement in the body stance. This will be more noticeable, of course, if the posture had been very poor but in most cases some improvement will be noticed.

It is a good plan after a week or so of the exercise to try the mirror test again and see if any improvement can be noted. This is often worthwhile as such an improvement will act as a stimulus to fresh effort, and also help one to concentrate on the parts of the body which need correction. As these exercises will definitely improve the posture, and incidentally help to normalise the spinal discs, another test will help to show how much has been gained, and especially whether the head and the neck structures are in balance. After finishing the last exercise and without trying to hold the body in any particular position, place a fairly heavy book on the top of the head. In order to balance the book the neck muscles will adjust the head to the position in which it should normally be held. If there is a tendency for the chin to be held too high the book will slide off so that the chin must be positioned to restore the balance and this is how the chin should be placed when standing in the ordinary way.

The proper posture of the neck is very important and efforts must be made to restore it if it has been lost. While people often think only about the lower back when the word disc is mentioned, the discs of the upper spine are just as important. When these discs are injured or under strain they give rise to many painful and discomforting symptoms, from headache to neuritis in the shoulders, arms and hands. To make sure that the head is balanced properly on the top of the spine and that the muscles of the neck are working in uniformity is the best way of countering disc troubles in the neck and by improving the posture of the whole body the task of the neck muscles are considerably reduced.

After these exercises have been performed for a week or two the muscles of the whole body will have become accustomed to their new tasks, and the spine, in particular, will have benefitted by having its structures, including the spinal discs, stretched and activated, and the individual should then pass on to the next series of testing exercises. As with the first series they are designed to see how the muscles and other parts of the system, particularly the spine, respond to movement, and here, again, it is insisted that graduation be the governing factor. They are based on the idea that you have to learn to walk before you can run, both of which demand the use of muscles and joints.

Exercise 7. Stand in your normal upright position, hands at side, with feet together and pointing directly ahead. Now in the most relaxed way lean over as if you are going to touch the floor with your finger tips. Do not do what so many people try to do : force your hands down to the floor. Simply let the whole body relax and let the amount of relaxation achieved be responsible for the lowering of your hands. What you will feel will be the strain of the hamstring muscles of your legs and these will be the limiting factor. You may notice that one hand may reach down farther than the other and this may be because there is an unevenness of the pull of the guy rope muscles of the spine, due most likely to a tilted position of it. Correct it by evening up the hands. After the body has been thoroughly relaxed in this position, first press one hand lower than the other and then follow with the other hand. In short, move the hands

D

up and down thus rotating the spine at the same time. A good
deal of time and thought should be spent doing this exercise
properly because it is a most valuable way of resting all the
muscles of the spine and at the same time taking the strain
off the spinal discs. A word or two of caution about it. The
head is held low and this may increase the blood flow to it;
in young people this may not be important and they can
maintain this position for some time. But with middle-aged and
older people it may be much more difficult for them to assume
this position and they should bear this in mind. Remember that it is a testing exercise, in that one attempts
to perform it but does not try to force oneself to its
full completion; one should also remember that whether the
hands touch the floor or not is more a matter of the build of
the patient rather than just flexibility. In some people the
ligaments involved are much longer and touching the toes or
the floor is very easily accomplished. We repeat, it is relaxation of the muscles and not forcing them that is the keynote of
this exercise.

Exercise 8. Lie flat on your abdomen on the floor, with
your arms tucked under your forehead. Before doing this
place a cushion on the floor in a position so that it will support the lower abdomen and the pelvic area. Relax the whole
body in this position for a few minutes, then stretch the legs
as much as possible. This puts quite a strain on the muscles of
the lower back and many will find this testing movement very
difficult to perform. One can be sure that when it is almost
impossible for the individual to do this that the spinal structures have been neglected and very much in need of restorative
exercises. Strength will come to these muscles only after a
certain amount of training so that at first no undue strain
must be used to perform this movement. As time goes by
and other exercises have been performed, one may return
to this particular one to see what progress has been made.
Weakness in this part of the back is often responsible for the
aching discomfort that many feel when they have been standing for a prolonged period, and also for the weak and tired
feeling in the back that may be experienced when rising in

the morning. This weakness of the lower back muscles will be a very real factor in the development of disc troubles since these structures will not be properly reinforced by strong supporting muscles and any slightly awkward movement of the body may strain the joints of the lumbar region. The muscles, discs and other structures of this part of the back have a great deal to do with weight-bearing and when they are weak the poor support of the spine gives rise to the dull aching pain that usually precedes disc and other back complaints.

Exercise 9. With hands behind your head adopt the same position, the cushion under the abdomen. Now attempt to lift up the upper part of the body; this will be easier if a weight is placed on the feet or if they are inserted under a heavy object. Here, again this is a real test for back muscles that are so often neglected. But for some people this is a straining movement and must be carefully performed. The older you are the more difficult it will be, and the less active exercise that you have taken will be shown in your inability to do this movement. After you have attempted to do this exercise with the hands behind the head, vary it by resting on the elbows and do a rocking movement, first raising the head and then the feet. If the cushion is made of foam rubber it will give a spring to the whole movement. This is a much easier movement to perform but quite valuable for the testing and strengthening of the muscles of the back. One should remember that so much time is spent with the body held in flexion, that when one has grown older the muscles which extend the body are almost out of use. The spinal discs can only retain their shape and size when they are constantly used, and if the body is practically always bent forward the discs will change to meet the weight-bearing. It is important, therefore, to counteract the effects of such habits and this kind of exercise, which puts the body, and the spine, in particular, into extension will have a rejuvenating effect upon those muscles which have been so long neglected. When it is said that people are as old as their spines, it means that they have failed to keep the spines flexible, and, without flexibility, the muscles and the discs will gradually lose their important functions. Growing old usually means growing bent as anyone can see from his fellow creatures.

Exercise 10. Lie on your back on the floor and allow yourself to relax for a few minutes, breathing in and out rhythmically. Place your hands on the lower abdomen and hold them firmly there. Now extend the legs out straight, keeping them together, and then raise them, or attempt to raise them, to about 8 to 12 inches off the floor. Hold them there until you count about five. If you have good muscles of the abdomen and the hips this movement may present no difficulty; on the contrary, weak muscles of those parts may make the movement too difficult. You will notice that under the pressure of the hands the abdominal muscles will tighten up, even if you only make the attempt to lift the legs, and do not succeed. To contract these muscles in that way is the first step towards the toning up of the muscles, and if you exercise them for a while in this way the added strength will enable you to complete the movement. The development of the abdominal muscles is very important in the acquisition of a good posture because if they are allowed to lose their tone and to sag they will place a great strain on the lower part of the spine. This may be an unsuspected cause of backache in many people and should be thought about in every case. Incidentally, weak abdominal muscles may be associated with complaints like constipation and hernia and a sound abdominal muscular system is a real preventive in this respect. This is a testing movement that should be applied to everyone suffering from any kind of backache, especially when there is a risk of disc troubles developing. An important point to bear in mind is that the legs must not be jerked up, nor must they be taken up more than a few inches; the lift must be a slow and deliberate one with the emphasis placed on the contraction of the abdominal muscles.

Exercise 11. Lie on the back on the floor with the hands pressed on the abdomen. The feet should have a weight on them or be hooked under a heavy piece of furniture. The idea is now to use the abdominal muscles to bring the body to the sitting-up position. The movement must not be jerky but made slowly and deliberately with the mind fixed on the abdominal muscles. As with the previous exercise, as soon as the attempt is made to perform it, the abdominal muscles will contract and this can be felt under the hands. Where there is not enough strength to do the full movement, enough of it may be done to bring the muscles into contraction and it will be found that after doing this a few times the full movement will be possible. In doing this exercise the hip muscles as well as the abdominal ones are used and this makes it a very valuable one. You may vary this exercise when it becomes too easy to accomplish by twisting the body first one side and then to the other as the body comes into the sitting-up position. This will help to develop the oblique muscles of the body, the ones placed at the sides of the body and attached to the ribs. Older people who have sagging abdominal muscles, and a weak and rigid spine that usually go with them, will find this rather a difficult exercise to perform and they should at first be cautious in attempting it. It is a testing exercise that will reveal many weaknesses of the muscular system, and one may be sure that until such weaknesses are overcome, bodily health and resistance cannot be at its highest standard.

The foregoing testing exercises should be carefully practised for a week or two, and during the time they are being used the weak parts of the system should be noted and attention paid to their eradication. The necessity for this kind of physical training is largely due to the fact that so many are confined to an urban life and are unable to get the exercise which is essential to bodily fitness. The various means of transport precludes the use of the limbs in natural exercise; on all sides we see the use of labour saving appliances and in every way the body is deprived of natural exercise. The result is that many people are suffering from many complaints that are due to under-use of their muscles and joints. Medical authorities attribute various complaints like headache, backache, and many other of the less serious illnesses to a lack of muscular exercise, while it is common knowledge that even serious diseases like peptic ulcers and heart disease is thought, by some authorities, to be related to occupations that are of a sedentary nature.

It is interesting to reflect on the fact that people are not, as a rule, put through tests to find out the weakness or otherwise of their muscles and joints. The heart may be examined, lungs X-rayed and other tests may be made, but it would be thought to be a departure from the ordinary examination if the muscular system and the joints were tested for mobility and efficiency. Yet there is no doubt at all that if this were done thoroughly it would reveal signs of weakness that if caught in time might prevent a great deal of trouble later on. For that reason we insist that the programme of exercises which we have outlined, if used intelligently, will prove a valuable way of estimating muscular and joint deficiencies, particularly of the spinal joints, a valuable safeguard against the disc troubles that are so much a feature of the present time. A test in time will save a lot of trouble in the future, and it will make you aware of weaknesses that you yourself will be able to overcome.

Exercise in Rheumatism and Arthritis

It is well-known that there is a close connection between disc troubles and rheumatism and arthritis. It is also well known, of course, that both diseases, although they are the oldest known to medical science, are still unsolved problems so far as cause and cure are concerned. Both of them are conditions which affect the structures of the body such as the muscles, ligaments and joints, so that it would be natural to expect that when there is a breakdown in the spinal discs the rheumatic and arthritic disease might well be an important factor. We stress these points in order to show that it is vitally important to do everything possible to keep the muscles and joints in working condition so as to offer as much resistance as we can to these diseases.

The point that should be stressed here is that the same factors which will help to preserve the full function and integrity of the spinal discs will also help to preserve the system from the ravages of these diseases. From this standpoint we should regard a better understanding of body mechanics to be a valuable asset both in the prevention of disc troubles and rheumatic and arthritic complaints. As we have already pointed out disc troubles are mainly brought about by strain, injury and bad posture, and when a joint and its surrounding structures have suffered in this way, the way is clearly open for rheumatism and arthritis to develop. Such a joint becomes a focal point for these diseases. If these diseases are due, as so many authorities think, to toxic or infectious substances circulating in the system then the weakened joint and its surrounding tissues is a very likely medium for further development of these troubles.

It follows that the removal of the same factors which lead to rheumatism and arthritis lead also to disc troubles so that in tackling the one we are preventing or at least mitigating the other. Also that when a person is suffering from one of these complaints, he or she must be on the lookout for back and disc trouble and must endeavour to keep all the susceptible joints in the body in as healthy condition as possible so as to prevent further deterioration. Indeed, one might go further and suggest that where rheumatism and arthritis appear to be a family weakness the possibility of susceptibility to disc troubles should always be considered.

What this means in practical terms for the individual is that any form of exercise that keeps the joint structures in a healthy condition is a worthwhile form of treatment in rheumatism and arthritis. What is still more important, perhaps, is that, even when these complaints are established, there is good reason to believe that exercise is one of the best ways of preventing further development. The same applies to postural adjustment. Whatever can be done to improve the posture of the body will be a most useful aid in the management of these complaints, since by taking the strain off the spine and other parts of the body it will activate their normal functions and thus increase their resistance to disease.

The proper posture of the body which is so bound up with the structures and mechanics of the spine, is much more a determinant of health and disease than many people imagine. Poor posture not only interferes with the body as an efficient instrument but it also affects all the vital organs as well. For example it cramps the chest and interferes with the breathing capacity; it depletes the nervous system by over-taxing the anti-gravity muscles, that help to maintain the erect position of the body, it tends to depress the organs in the digestive tract and the pelvis, and it impedes normal circulation. No system can work efficiently under such circumstances, and, in time, the general health and resistance of the body must suffer. Lowering the health potential in this way is an invitation to trouble, and if there should be a tendency in the system to rheumatism and arthritis this is a very good way of allowing it to get a foothold.

Whatever other measures may be adopted for the treatment of these complaints, there is no doubt that properly planned exercise should be an essential part of them. It is the only way by which we can keep the discs, the muscles and the joints in normal condition and for that reason the testing exercises should form a part of the measures which every sufferer from rheumatism and arthritis should adopt. As we have shown, these sufferers are potential victims of the disc lesions and they cannot afford to run the risk of a breakdown because every affected joint is a further link in the chain of disease.

Exercise After Injuries

Few people are likely to go through life without some injury to the back which may involve the spinal discs. Apart from accidents such as falls and car injuries, young people often injure the spine in the various games and sports. It may be serious enough to need medical attendance or it may only be some kind of muscle strain that the individual feels will put itself right by rest. In the very early stages of the trouble this may well be true, but as soon as the acute pain has subsided it is very important to make quite sure that the injured muscles and joints have fully recovered their normal function and to do this it will be necessary to use the testing exercises. It should be pointed out that pain is the important guide when doing such exercises. It often happens that the muscles and the joints may be very stiff after an injury and the sufferer may be afraid of exercising the parts. But so long as it can be done with the minimum of pain no danger is involved. Indeed, all the stiffness must be overcome by exercise before one can truly consider that the parts are back to normal. The discs, in particular, may suffer if the limitation in the muscles and joints is allowed to remain, as movement is vital to them. In addition, one must remember that any kind of stiffness in muscles and joints will interfere with the circulation of the blood and lymph, which, in turn, will deprive the tissues of the essential nutrients.

Gaining Muscular Control

One of the differences between exercise that comes as a result of working and that which is done for the express purpose of building up muscular tone and strength is the use of the mind. In the former case the mind is on the work in hand. The manual worker is not concentrating his mind on his own muscles when he is doing his job; the strength and development of his muscular system is quite incidental to him. With the use of exercise for treatment purposes such as we are discussing here in relation to disc troubles, the position is quite different. It is all important that the mind be focussed on the parts of the body to be affected, and if this is done with studied concentration definite muscular control will be gained. This is a very important aspect of the subject, and one which the individual should very carefully observe. For that reason exercise, to be really effective as a treatment measure, must be carried out with the purpose for which it is aimed, firmly fixed in the mind. That is one of the reasons why testing exercises in which the person is trying to assess the condition of the various muscles and joints, and the flexibility of the spine, are likely to be of far greater value than those which are performed with very little concern as to what the effects of them will be; and it is interesting to note that when control over the muscles has been gained in this way it will be possible to make the excercises much more effective with the expenditure of less time and less energy.

CHAPTER SEVEN

GENERAL CONSIDERATIONS

In all troubles affecting the muscular system, joints and cartilages we may be quite sure that tension is an accompanying condition. Unrelieved tension causes a great drain on the nervous system and may be regarded as one of the real problems of modern life with the mental and emotional strains which it places upon the majority of people. What we should bear in mind is that when tension exists it does so because there is no available outlet for the pent up nervous or mental energy, and that while this condition continues the whole system cannot operate efficiently. Tension leads to many symptoms, especially in the muscular system, where we may find tender spots and minor aches and pains. When the parts are under tension in this way it will interfere with normal function and this is especially true of the spine. In some instances the muscles will be in a state of contraction and this may impose strains upon the other structures, particularly the discs. It has been recognised that a condition such as this may well be a precursor of a breakdown in the disc, or discs, and it should always be regarded as a warning signal.

Tension is a reaction of the bodily system through the muscles, and we may be quite sure that when it occurs, there is some explosive energy within it that needs to be released. Its natural release is through exercise of some kind. In earlier times when life was lived through conditions and occupations that called all the muscles into use there was no real problem about it. But under modern conditions, very few people are engaged in occupations that use up their physical energy, and hence their tensions and the ailments that derive from them.

Tension uses up nervous energy without assisting the normal functions of the system; it has an adverse effect upon the circulation, and may predispose to variations in blood pressure; it dissipates energy that should be employed in the elimination processes and it acts as an irritant in a vicious circle between mind and body. It is, of course, antagonistic to true rest and relaxation. Tension is often regarded as the scourge of modern day living and many blame it for the excessive amount of drugs that are in use at the present time.

The real release for tension can come only from exercise, the vigorous use of the muscles. Many people are under the impression that the answer to it lies in relaxation but the truth of the matter is that relaxation should always be secondary to exercise. The body should be used sufficiently enough to tire the muscles so that there is a natural desire to rest and relax. To try to relax the body without taking into consideration this important fact is to court disappointment. Exercise relieves the tension and then relaxation will follow.

The same is true of breathing and this is a very important subject when considered in connection with exercise. To practise deep breathing when the system is in no need of extra oxygen is mostly a waste of time and effort. The natural need for fuller breathing can only be brought about by exercise of some kind. Then, when the oxygen is being used up, there will be a demand for deeper breathing to satisfy that need, and it is at that time that it will bring the greatest benefit to the body.

It is very important that these facts about tension, exercise, relaxation and breathing should be kept in mind when using special movements as preventive measures in disc troubles. To get the best results from exercise we must work in accord with the best interests of the body.

Corrective Exercises

If the reader has used the mirror test and gone through the testing exercises he will now be in a position to estimate his own particular spinal weaknesses, and able also to gauge his muscular condition. If the exercises have been performed regularly there will be no doubt that a general improvement will have been noticed, but it may be that there may still remain certain defects in the posture and body mechanics that may need correction. And in this section we plan to provide special instruction whereby he will be able to rectify them.

It is most likely that these weaknesses may be seen in the curves of the spine and departures from their normal lines, and sometimes it is necessary to apply movements to them for specific purposes. For example, we may get a curve in which the spine seems to be tilted from the base or we may get a slight double curve. In this strict sense of the term, as it is ordinarily applied, curve is rather a strong one to use; a slight variation in the upward line might be a better description. But where such a condition exists it does emphasise a weakness and if it can be corrected there will be far less likelihood of disc trouble.

Lumbar Region. Exercise 12.

Sometimes the spine in this area is curved sideways and this means that the muscle on the one side of the spine will be shortened while on the other it will be lengthened. This can be greatly helped by side-bending exercise. Stand with feet apart. Place the hands on the sides of the body just at the lower ribs, fingers pointing to the back. Now bend over as far as possible to one side pressing inward with the hand on that side. Then do the same to the other side. In this way the muscles are thoroughly stretched and if the exercise is done carefully one can tell which side needs the more vigorous stretching. Follow this up by dropping the hands to the sides and then, pressing one hand on the outer side of the leg, reach down with it as far as possible. Repeat with the other hand. These movements will even up the pull of the back muscles and improve the balance of the spine.

Dorsal Region. Exercise 13.

In this region the ribs support the spine so that there is less likelihood of much of a curve, but it is helpful to have it in mind if the shoulders are uneven. The shoulders will be higher on one side than the other, and so sidebend to lower the higher shoulder, and, at the same time, reach above the head with the hand on the other side. This will help to lift up the ribs and loosen their joints where they are attached to the spine. A tendency to a curve in this area of the spine depresses the rib joints on one side and many aches and pains may arise, unsuspectedly, from this source.

Neck Region. Exercise 14.

In many ways the neck is the most vulnerable part of the spine, and because of its mobility it is constantly subjected to jolts and strains. It has to carry the weight of the head which weighs about 15 lbs., and it has to compensate for defects in the basic posture. For that reason it is liable to suffer from muscular and nervous tensions and many people complain of neck aches and pains. Every effort, therefore, should be made to keep the head well balanced and the neck muscles in good tone Sight and hearing depend, in some measure, on the condition of the neck which should be strong yet flexible.

Because the neck may lose its freedom of movement it should be exercised every day. It should be moved forward as far as possible and backward in the same way. Then bend the head sideways; this is a very important movement because the neck is often limited in this movement. Then rotate the head as much as possible. By doing these exercises daily one is making sure that the discs of the upper spine are being used as they should be, and this will go a long way to preventing them from thinning and getting out of shape; when one sees the people around with surgical collars one may be sure that these exercises were neglected. In addition to this, there are very important nerves and blood vessels passing through the neck region upon which the circulation of the brain depends.

Time spent in making sure that the posture of the neck is properly adjusted is time well spent. As people grow older there is a tendency for them to carry the neck too far ahead, as it were. To prevent this the following exercise will help:

Exercise 15. Hold the body as still as possible and then push the neck as far forward as possible and then as far backward as possible. Then get into the habit during the day to tuck the chin down in towards the chest. If the muscles of the neck are weak they may be strengthened by placing a towel at the back of the head and neck and holding it in front with both hands. Then press the head against the towel and resist with the neck muscles. This exercise should be done if there is pain in the shoulders because it usually arises from a weakness of the upper spine.

Rounded Shoulders. Exercise 16.

When the curves of the spine are too deep they promote the rounded-shoulder type of body. If this is allowed to go on the real danger is not so much in the shoulder region but in the curves themselves, although rounded shoulders do tend to cramp the chest. If the curves are not reduced the danger is that the discs in the curves will alter their shape and the curve of the spine will become fixed, with perhaps arthritic changes taking place later on. The best excercise for correction is what has sometimes been called the 'lazy-man's' excercise. It means lying flat on a hard carpeted floor with the arms stretched out horizontally. If this position is held for a while the spine tends to flatten itself out on the floor, and thus to reduce the curves. When there is a deep curve in the lumbar region the flat position may cause pain in that region. To relieve this draw the feet up to the buttocks and relieve the strain and then straighten them out again.

People of middle and later age, who have developed deep curves in the spine, may find this a very strenuous exercise and it should then be done with caution. When the curves in the spine are very deep it is very difficult for the whole spine to flatten out and in some cases the body rests on the buttocks, the shoulders and the top of the head, with space between the lumbar region, the neck region and the floor. When the curve is very deep in the neck there is a tendency for the top rather than the back of the head to rest on the floor. The progress made by the exercise can be measured by the contact which the whole of the spine makes with the floor.

In certain cases the reverse is true. Then the spine is too

straight or curved outwards. The position to correct this is to lie on the abdomen and then raise the body by pressing up with the arms at the same time holding the lower part of the abdomen on the floor. This tends to deepen the curve in the lower back. This position will be found to give grateful relief if the individual has been standing for a prolonged period.

Exercises for Spinal Rotation. Exercise 17.

The muscles of the back that are generally neglected in exercise are the ones that rotate the spine. The muscles that are used in the forward and backward movements of the body get a fair amount of use in daily occupation and they are usually pretty well attended to in the various systems of exercise. In consequence the rotating muscles may be weak and therefore more liable to strain. In this respect, it is interesting to notice that it is, generally speaking, in the rotating or side-bending movements of the spine, that the damage to the discs often occur. It is wise to bear this fact in mind, and to make as sure as one can that these muscles are toned up by suitable exercise.

Leg movements may be used to stimulate the muscles of rotation. For example, lie flat on the back with the arms extended level with the shoulders. Raise one leg keeping it as straight as possible. Now allow it to fall across the body until it reaches the floor on that side. At the same time maintain a firm position with the shoulders and arms. Repeat with the other leg. This exercise will tone up the muscles in the lumbar region. This exercise can be modified in this way: Still flat on the back with arms extended. Bring feet up to the buttocks, keeping them flat on the floor. Now bend both knees over to the one side as far as possible and then to the other side. The shoulders and arms are kept firmly on the floor.

A final variation of this exercise is as follows : Same position with knees bent and feet as near the buttocks as possible. Lace the fingers, holding the arms straight up in the air. Now bend as far as possible with the arms over to one side and at the same time bend the knees in the opposite direction. This is a splendid stretching movement that will stimulate the muscles in those backs that are often neglected.

Exercise for Pelvis and Hips. Exercise 18.

The spine is set on the pelvis and the big muscles supporting it arise therefrom. The great muscles of the legs are also attached to the pelvis so that there is a constant interplay of forces placing on this part of the body a great deal of strain. The weight of the upper body is transmitted through the pelvis to the hips, legs, and the sacro-iliac joints which, although bound together with powerful ligaments, have to take up considerable strain. As these structures form the foundation of the spinal column it is not surprising that maladjustment of these should upset the balance of the spine. Today many people hear of the occurrence of sacro-iliac lesions, and it is unfortunately true that where these exist much of the compensating balance will take place in the spine above, which will place other spinal discs at risk.

Attention should, therefore, be paid to the pelvis and the hips to make quite sure that they are functioning normally, and the following exercise will be found most valuable in that respect. It will help to mobilize the muscles of the region so that there will be a good balance between them with the weight of the body properly distributed through the hips.

Stand with one foot on a book or an object that is about 2 to 3 inches in thickness. Now holding both legs quite stiff, try to reach the floor with the other foot that is free. Then lift the foot as high as possible and repeat. Do the same with the other leg. If this movement is done properly the effect of it will be felt across the lower back, and if it is persisted in, it will loosen up the joints of this area and make a real improvement in body posture. The exercise can be varied by standing with both feet on the floor and then keeping both legs quite stiff raise one then the other. The lifting power comes from the pelvic and buttock area. This exercise should be done by those who have weak pelvic or sacro-iliac joints.

Exercise for the Feet

It may be rather difficult for some people to realise the connection between the feet and the spinal discs; even when they may have suffered from disc lesions the connection may have never crossed their minds, but if we think about it for a few minutes we shall soon see that it is a fact that should not be overlooked. The feet carry the weight of the whole body and it should be equally distributed between the two of them. Defects in the posture may disturb these weight-bearing functions and more weight may fall on one foot than the other. This may tend to weaken the arch of the foot and in the long run, the spinal discs may be affected by the changed position of the spine.

Another important function of the foot is its shock-absorbing capacity, which depends, of course, upon the spring-like action of the inside of the foot. If the foot is rigid, or if the arch has fallen, the foot will be unable to absorb the shock which it experiences in walking, running, jumping and so on, and then the shocks may be transferred to the spine where their effects will have to be dealt with by the spinal discs. But when the foot is flexible, and its arch spring-like in its actions the spine may be spared these shocks with real gain by the nervous system.

For these reasons it is very important to keep the muscles of the feet strong and toned up which means that they should be regularly exercised. In some ways the feet are the most abused parts of our bodies, they are enclosed in shoes, and are, to a great extent, deprived of unfettered movement. This must, of course, interfere with the normal circulation, and it is surprising that more people do not suffer from foot troubles than they do.

If there is some disparity between the arches of the feet this should be regarded as a potential danger for the back and the spine and it should be rectified. This may, of course, be beyond the individual's own power, but it will be up to him to perform the necessary exercises to keep the structures of the feet in good condition.

Exercise 19. The shoes should be removed when doing exercises. The old fashioned idea of raising the body on the toes is a very good start and it should

E

be done until there is a feeling of tiredness in the muscles. Vary this by standing on a thick book, or a suitable object, and try to reach the ground with the toes, spreading them out as much as possible when doing so. Then sit on a chair and move the feet up and down, stretching them as much as you can. Then rotate them at the ankle joints. These movements will increase the circulation and tone up the muscles.

People who stand for long periods during the day may suffer from swollen feet in the evenings and this puffiness will weaken the muscles and arches. Before doing the exercises it is a good plan to lie on the back on the floor and rest the feet on a wall, placing them as high as possible above the body. This will reduce the swelling and relax the feet. As a matter of fact, when the feet are tired, and, perhaps, suffering from tension this position will be found to be very relieving.

A word or two should be said about footwear. The very high heels that are worn by some women are potentially dangerous so far as the discs of the spine are concerned. Elevating the heel in that manner must be compensated for in the weight carrying functions of the body, and it is the spine that will have to bear the burden. This will result in backache of varying degree, and if this is allowed to persist for any length of time, we may be sure that changes will take place in the spinal discs that will lead to many other troubles in later life. The same is true when the feet and the toes are cramped in pointed shoes. This is bound to interfere with the weight carrying function of the feet, and in time will affect the posture of the body. The development of bunions follow the use of narrow and pointed shoes which is a very expensive price to pay for such a fashion. When bunions become painful ones whole gait may be altered and this may well be an important factor in the making of disc troubles.

People who live in towns and have to walk on hard pavements should use rubber on the heels of the shoes. This will help to break the shock of the impact on the hard surface of the streets. Some men, in trying, no doubt, to economise, sometimes use steel tips on the heels of the shoes but this is a false economy because it does not help to prevent shock to the feet and the spine. Men's shoes, as a rule, are better designed to meet the natural needs of the feet, but there has been a tendency of recent years for the pointed shoe to become the fashion. It was recently reported that men are developing bunions in increasing numbers and this may be the result of the present fashion.

General Body Conditioning

While special exercises are often required for the correction of specific conditions, such as disc troubles, we should not forget that the whole body works as a unit and that the general state of the system is always important. While we can do so much good by means of the exercise that is done as physical training, the general exercise that is taken in the form of walking, hiking, cycling and other outdoor recreational pursuits, is invaluable in keeping the body in its best shape. In addition, of course, there is the added value of fresh air and as these activities generally tend to take one away from the less pure atmosphere of the towns and cities we gain in that way also.

Vigorous walking is one of the best forms of natural exercise; it speeds up the circulation and gets rid of the waste products of the tissues. But to do it properly the body must be in good condition, and it is particularly important that the feet be suitably clad and prepared for the task. Walking with feet that tend to make it a burden will deprive the exercise of most of its value. In such a case the care of the feet along the lines we have already suggested will make walking more pleasurable and more profitable.

Gardening is another activity that takes people into the fresh air and helps to keep the system in good general condition, but it should be borne in mind that there is a strong tendency for the back to be constantly bending and the weekend gardener, as we have already said, may make himself a candidate for disc troubles. For that reason a few minutes spent, after a session in the garden, relaxing the back muscles will often avoid a good deal of future trouble.

Over-exertion in these activities is to be avoided, especially if one is not in tip top shape, and it is far better to do too little than to do too much and suffer a breakdown. It is far easier to prevent such troubles by a little foresight than to rectify them afterwards. This is said, out of the experience of having known of a great many cases of spinal disc troubles arising as a result of injudicious outdoor activities, that carried an ill-trained body beyond its ordinary capacities.

Overweight and Disc Troubles

Overweight of the body, or obesity, is becoming a major problem in many civilised countries. Authorities associate it with many serious diseases such as diabetes and coronary breakdown, and it is certainly a serious factor in the various complaints affecting the muscles, joints and discs of the spine. It is true, of course, that overweight is allied to the nutrition of the body and that careful attention must be paid to diet if the complaint is to be controlled. It is so easy at the present time to get an abundance of foods that are rich in starch and sugar, and these are the articles of diet that add the fat to the tissues.

Overweight may contribute to disc troubles in two ways: first, by adding to the body weight and thus imposing great strain on the spinal discs, and secondly, by weakening the muscular system and undermining the supporting structures of the body. It is easy to imagine the strain imposed upon the discs, in their weight-bearing function, when the body weight is increased, as it may be, by, say 40 or 50 lbs or more. The whole spine will be under constant strain in carrying out the daily tasks and going up and down steps, where the body's balancing mechanism is brought into play, make the movements of the spinal joints very difficult.

Overweight also interferes with the supporting qualities of the muscles. The spinal column is particularly dependent upon the strength of the muscles, which act as guy ropes to it, and any failure on their part in this respect is a direct incitement to disc trouble. Instead of being in good tone, and responsive to every action to which the spine is subject, the muscles are sluggish and slow of reaction. This places the discs in a precarious position, with every movement of the body liable to put them at risk. And to make things even more difficult for the supporting qualities of the muscles of the spine and the spinal discs, the overweight person develops a heavy sagging abdomen which directly pulls on the back and adds to its burden.

Overweight cannot be managed without some regulation of the appetite and the amount and quality of the food that is consumed, which, in many cases, means in some ways having to live with a certain amount of hunger. One has only to look through the various advertisements in all kinds of journals to see what a problem overweight is for some people and the hundred and one different modes of attack that are suggested as ways of combating it.

To a great extent it has coincided with the present method of living, where while food is plentiful, physical exercise is at a low ebb. The less strenuous work becomes and the more people are disinclined to rectify this by exercise, the more people are likely to suffer from this disability. While it is true to say that the regulation of food intake is of major importance, there is no doubt that a great deal can be done to mitigate the effects of obesity by keeping up regular and fairly vigorous exercise. In any case, so far as the condition of the spinal discs are concerned it is vital that the muscles be kept free of fatty tissue; this is the main point at issue. If a full intake of food simply means that more and healthy muscle is developed from it, then no great harm will accrue. It is the accumulation of fat that makes obesity perilous and exercise is the best way of breaking it down in the tissues and getting rid of it that way. Without exercise it permeates all the muscles, including those of the heart and spine, and these are the vital parts of the system where it can do most harm.

If one has to choose between a strictly limited diet and little exercise, and a normal one, with plenty of exercise, the latter is by far the better plan. It is the safer one so far as the health and resistance of the body is concerned, and, especially so, with regard to the integrity of the muscles, joints and cartilages of the system.

Disc Troubles and Young People

Many years ago it used to be thought that the aching back,

which was associated with lumbago and sciatica was very much the burden of the older person, but, today, it is not unusual to find the condition in quite young people of both sexes. Even adolescents are not exempt, and it is, therefore, a problem that may have to be faced quite early in life. It is not easy, perhaps, to be quite sure why this is so, but it may be that young people seem to grow more quickly, that, as a rule, they are fed to the point of putting on too much fat, and that the foods that are most easily obtained, such as the refined foods, predispose to a certain weakness of the body structures, especially the spinal discs.

The world has changed radically for young people. It is not so long ago that they had to be more active; they had not the things they have today that tend to make them lead a more sedentary life. The motor car, television and so on, all these things predispose to physical inactivity. They may sit for hours at their desks in schools; spurts of strenuous activity will not make up for long hours of sitting around; And if the spurts come without preparation they may have the effect of catching the weak muscles off guard producing, what the advisers may call a 'slipped disc', a very troublesome complaint at such a time.

In youth, the spinal discs, like all the other parts of the body, are in the developmental stage. At that stage they are supplied with blood vessels and have a fuller content of water than in later life. They are, of course, very resilient, allowing greater freedom of movement than in later life. The muscles, too, are quickly developing as the body is changing to meet the needs of adult life. In the ordinary way, of course, Nature takes care of these things and the individual has little to bother about. But there are times when attention is required to make sure that development is proceeding normally and this is true, in particular, of the spinal column which in youth may be subject to habits and strains that will be detrimental in later life if they pass unnoticed.

More attention should be paid to the back and spine in young people. Outbursts of energy and activity may produce minor disabilities in the spine that, unless they are corrected, may be real defects when adult life is reached. Well directed exercise is the answer. It would be a good thing if young people could be persuaded to use the testing exercises to evaluate the strength of their muscles, especially those of the spine, so that if there were signs of weakness they could be rectified. In youth there is the real advantage of being able to constructively influence the development of the body, and minor defects that would be resistant to treatment in later life can be overcome when the body is young.

The best time for the prevention of disc troubles is in youth and the sooner this fact is recognised the sooner we shall be able to reduce the number of weak and ailing backs that plague the life of so many adults at the present time. For in spite of the fact that these troubles seem to arise without warning, and without any good reason, the plain fact is that they are the culmination of a series of events in which the body has steadily moved towards a crisis. When this occurs we are apt to concentrate all our thoughts on the present and the future and conveniently ignore the past.

Fibrositis and Disc Troubles

The term fibrositis is often used when a person suffers from vague muscular pains, especially those which seem to resemble some kind of rheumatism. The term 'Fibrositis' is clearly just a term of convenience since it has no precise definition. Literally it means inflammation of fibres, but that gives one very little idea as to what it is meant to convey. It may be a very real thing from the sufferer's point of view, having unpleasant symptoms such as pain in the muscles and very sensitive and tender areas in them. Recently, however, opinion has been coming round to the idea that these pains and tender muscles may be the result of nerve irritation caused by disorders of the spinal discs and the adjacent tissues.

The discs, as we know, are closely associated with the nerve roots that emerge from the spinal cord, and when they are under strain from muscle contraction or some form of postural maladjustment, these nerves are irritated and send their messages through the muscular tissues which they supply. If this is so, and there is plenty of evidence to show that it is supported by many authorities, then the simplest way to manage such ailments is to make sure that the normal functions of the spine are restored by improving the posture of the body and by improving body mechanics. In a word one should look with more questioning eyes toward the spine for a solution.

From this standpoint the testing exercises can be used to good effect. In this way one will be able to find out where there is tension in the spine, where the muscles are irritated, and then adopt the exercises most suitable for remedial action. In this sense the fibrositis may prove a blessing in disguise, since it may be the warning signal that the muscles of the back are under irritation and tension, and thus alert the person to the fact that unless preventive measures are taken, disc troubles of a more serious nature may follow.

The same reasoning applies to many forms of neuritis that afflict people in the various muscles of the body. While such ailments may appear to be of local origin many of them can be traced back to the spinal nerves, and some form of irritation affecting them. The fact that such pains may appear in parts remote from the spinal nerves, in, perhaps the hands or the feet, is simply evidence that the nerve fibres are found in every part of the system, and that nerve impulses which carry the sense of pain may pass from one part of the body to another. Although sciatica is felt in the leg and foot the origin of the pain is in the lower spinal nerves, and this applies to other forms of neuritis.

Faulty use of the body, with its interference with proper posture and body mechanics will invariably effect the joints of the spine, often producing neuritic symptoms in the muscles of the limbs. It is wise to look further than the local symptoms, and in such cases it is more than worthwhile to use the testing exercises to see if there are tensions and weaknesses in the spinal region that may be irritating the nerve trunks. As we have pointed out these symptoms may be the forerunner of disc troubles, which, if they are caught in the early stages, make the prevention of further deterioration possible.

Summing Up

There is no need to exaggerate the disc problem. Those who have suffered from it have good reason to know of its incapacitating effects, the seriousness of the pains, and the troubles which are involved in the treatment. Apart from the actual suffering, it may mean prolonged rest in bed, followed by various forms of treatment, and finish up with the wearing of some kind of corset. At worst it may mean surgical treatment. In many cases total recovery may not be achieved and the individual, if previously engaged on, comparatively speaking, heavy work, may have to change over to work of much lighter kind. In short, the effects of the disability may radically alter the individual's way of life and become a dominant factor influencing his future activities. There are, unfortunately, hundreds of people who find themselves in this kind of situation and, so far as the evidence goes, the trouble is on the increase involving perhaps a million or more people.

These, of course, represent the more serious cases. On the other hand, the minor troubles arising in this way, amount to many more. One authority went so far as to say that at some time in their lives every man, woman and child could expect to suffer from the so-called 'slipped disc' and while this is undoubtedly an exaggeration it does give one an idea of how many people are predisposed to this weakness. The reason for estimating the trouble at such a high level is probably due to the fact, that, whereas in the older days backache was attributed to many causes from colds, draughts and the kidneys, ('every picture tells a story' myth) at the present time practically every form of backache is considered to be the result of a disc lesion. In days gone by when children experienced vague pains in the limbs they were regarded as growing pains; today, they are far more likely to be attributed to irritation from the spinal discs. Certainly, when such pains occur in the adult the thought should, quite rightly, fly to that source.

No matter how effective any treatment may be for any disability there is no doubt that prevention is always better than cure. In cases where the spinal discs are involved, we have every reason to know that treatment is not always so effective and that the need for prevention is even more important. That is the aspect of the subject with which every person should be primarily concerned. This is true, of course, if he or she has never suffered from the trouble, and perhaps, even more true of those who have suffered and want to feel more secure for the future. There is no other complaint on which it is more important to place the emphasis on prevention, and as we have shown that prevention depends upon a better appreciation of the importance of body posture and body mechanics there is every reason to believe that it can be made really effective.

It is not always appreciated as much as it should be how dependent we are for our health and resistance to disease on the mechanical aspect of the body. People may think in terms of taking medicines for their complaints and do other things along such lines, but they rarely consider the human machine as an instrument that needs mechanical adjustment. Of course, this point of view has been emphasised by medical authorities from time to time, as witness this statement by Dr Goldthwait, one of the foremost authorities in the United States: 'An individual is in the best health only when the body is so used that there is no strain on any of its parts. This means that when standing the body is held fully erect, with no strain on the joints, bones, ligaments, muscles, or any other structures. There should be adequate room for all the viscera, so that their function can be performed normally.' A great Australian anatomist put it this way: 'If we exclude specific infectious diseases, which are in the main preventable and due to segregation, we may define health as a correlation of all the bodily systems to the erect posture, and ill-health as a failure of one or more systems to correlate to it.'

The prevalence of disc troubles is clear evidence that this important aspect of human well being has been sadly neglected in spite of the work which these two doctors did to emphasise the need for more attention to be paid to proper posture and of body mechanics. The spinal discs are undoubtedly the focal point for all the stresses and strains which faulty posture and wrong usage of the body imposes upon the human frame. When we see people working, playing, and generally lifting and moving about with no regard for these bodily principles we may be fairly sure that they are likely candidates for slipped or herniated discs and all the future difficulties that may portend.

It will be realised that so far as prevention is concerned it is not only a matter of exercise which must be used to strengthen the muscles and aid them in their supporting tasks; it is also a matter of developing better habits in adjusting the body mechanically to its daily tasks. In order to do this one must have some knowledge of the body and the way it works. It should be a part of our educational system to instil into childrens' minds the importance of the mechanical aspect of body usage, and help them to form good habits by sitting properly at their studies as well as doing physical exercise. This might spare them a lot of trouble when they become adults and have to meet modern day stresses and strains. If disc troubles go on increasing at the rate they have been doing in the last couple of decades, the teaching of good body mechanics will have to become more generally recognised by society as a necessary health measure, and to make this effective there will have to be co-operation in the homes and in the schools. Industry, too, should be interested, if only because of the fact that it stands to gain physical efficiency in its workers and a great decrease in the loss of working hours.

The prevention of disc troubles devolves, in the last analysis upon the individual, and although he may be in possession of such information as we have outlined in this book, it will avail him nothing if he does not do his part in putting it into practice. It cannot be repeated too often that there is no substitute for exercise, and only the individual can do it for himself. The same is true of forming good bodily habits, in standing, sitting, lifting and in all the hundred and one ways in which use is made of the body. No outsider can do these things for him, or indeed help him, if he has not the will and the persistence to do them for himself.

Résumé

Use the mirror test to get an idea of your posture and its shortcomings, if any.

Do the first set of testing exercises, noting any slight defects that need to be rectified.

Go gradually on to the other exercises, always remembering that when they are difficult to do care must be taken not to strain. If you do not succeed at first, try again later.

As you become aware of your weak points try to choose the movements which will help to strengthen them.

If the muscles feel fatigued after exercising drop them for a day or so. But when used to them do them regularly.

Use the mirror test from time to time to test improvement in your posture.

Exercise to strengthen your muscles but also to improve your posture.

Remember to use your body as correctly as possible when lifting and doing strenuous tasks.

Finally, do it now.

Fr. David Kalert, omi

Fr. David Kalert, OMI

P.S. If you can <u>renew your Association membership by May 1</u>, I would also like to send you a prayer card picturing the Icon of Our Lady of the Snows at the new Church of Our Lady of the Snows at the Shrine. <u>The card will be blessed at the May 5th dedication of the Church.</u>

Oblates of Mary Immaculate.

One of the over 5,000 Oblates who will be helped by your Association membership is Fr. Gene Prendiville, OMI, who represents a 50-year history of Oblate ministry to persons with profound disabilities at the Lincoln Development Center in Lincoln, Illinois. For five decades, Oblates have been bringing spiritual comfort to the profoundly disabled and their families ... not only in Lincoln, but also many similar facilities throughout the world. With major ministries in over 60 countries, the Oblates have a 165-year history of service to the neglected, poor, and unchurched. And throughout this long history, we have always reflected a desire to have lay

MISSIONARY OBLATES OF MARY IMMACULATE
National Shrine of Our Lady of the Snows — Belleville, IL 62223-4694

over please

EXERCISE INDEX

Carefully and without strain, do each of the following exercises, taking extra care where cautioned. Whenever you feel a movement is not easily accomplished, spend a minute or so concentrating on it.

Regular use of these exercises will pinpoint possible trouble areas, which when manipulated will become strengthened.

The region of the back affected by each exercise is indicated by the shaded area of the spine shown next to it.

EXERCISE 1

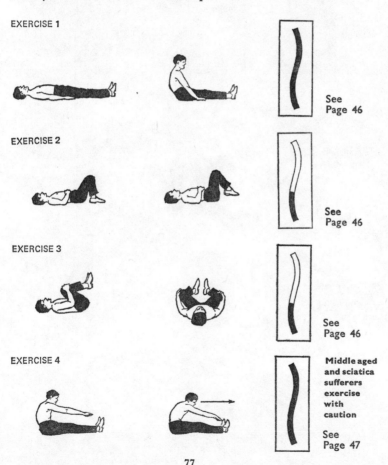

See
Page 46

EXERCISE 2

See
Page 46

EXERCISE 3

See
Page 46

EXERCISE 4

Middle aged
and sciatica
sufferers
exercise
with
caution

See
Page 47

77

EXERCISE 5

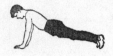

exercise
with
caution

See
Page 47

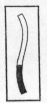

EXERCISE 6

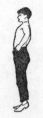

See
Page 47

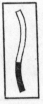

EXERCISE 7

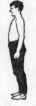 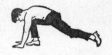

Middle aged
and over.
Beware of
faintness

See
Page 49

EXERCISE 8

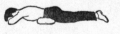

See
Page 50

EXERCISE 9

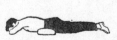 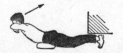

See
Page 51

EXERCISE 10

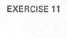
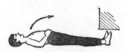
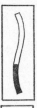

See
Page 52

EXERCISE 11

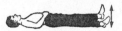

See
Page 52

EXERCISE 12

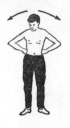
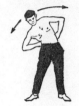
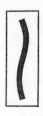

See
Page 60

EXERCISE 13

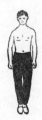
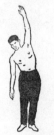
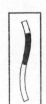

See
Page 60

EXERCISE 14

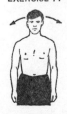
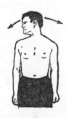
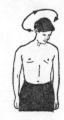
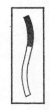

See
Page 62

EXERCISE 15

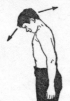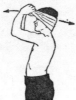

See
Page 61

EXERCISE 16

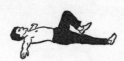

See
Page 62

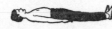

EXERCISE 17

See
Page 63

EXERCISE 18

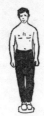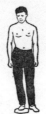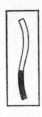

See
Page 64